Eczema Cure

Eczema No More - The Ultimate Guide to Knowing and Keeping Eczema Under Control

By

Fhilcar Faunillan

Fhilcar Faunillan

Eczema Cure

The information provided herein is stated to be truthful and consistent, in that any liability, in terms of inattention or otherwise, by any usage or abuse of any policies, processes, or directions contained within is the solitary and utter responsibility of the recipient reader. Under no circumstances will any legal responsibility or blame be held against the publisher for any reparation, damages, or monetary loss due to the information herein, either directly or indirectly.

Respective authors own all copyrights not held by the publisher.

The information herein is offered for informational purposes solely, and is universal as so. The presentation of the information is without contract or any type of guarantee assurance.

The trademarks that are used are without any consent, and the publication of the trademark is without permission or backing by the trademark owner. All trademarks and brands within this book are for clarifying purposes only and are the owned by the owners themselves, not affiliated with this document.

Table of Contents

INTRODUCTION

I want to thank you and congratulate you for downloading the book, *"Eczema Cure: Eczema No More – The Ultimate Guide to Knowing and Keeping Eczema Under Control"*.

This book contains proven steps and strategies on how to prevent the flaring-up and worsening of Eczema.

Health is pretty much what we all want to take care of nowadays. It drives us to work with the things we need to do and at the same time, help us enjoy through life. But despite all the efforts, some diseases can still affect us most especially when the causes are highly hereditary and under uncontrollable environments, one of these diseases is eczema.

Eczema is a common condition that starts early in childhood and continuously carried on through adolescence and even adulthood. There is no definite cause for this condition, however, there are a cluster of irritants that may trigger the flaring of eczema. These triggers may also differ among individuals, but nevertheless, preventive measures must be taken into action.

As of now, there is still no treatment that can totally eradicate eczema from one's system so that it would no longer affect people once they reach adulthood.What we have now are temporary treatments of eczema that can keep them under control.

If you are thinking how much these treatments would cost you, there is actually no need to worryfor you can actually make natural ointments out of the products that can simply be found in your gardens or kitchens.

What will you expect to get from reading this book? This will provide you with information about eczema—its symptoms, types, possible triggers, as well as prevalence among age groups, genders, and across races. Most of all, this book will provide you with preventive measures and possible natural treatments that are within your reach. Get ideas of what you can include when preparing for your food in order to avoid or hinder your present condition from getting worse.

Fhilcar Faunillan

Thanks again for downloading this book, I hope you enjoy it!

Chapter 1 - All About Eczema Symptoms And Types

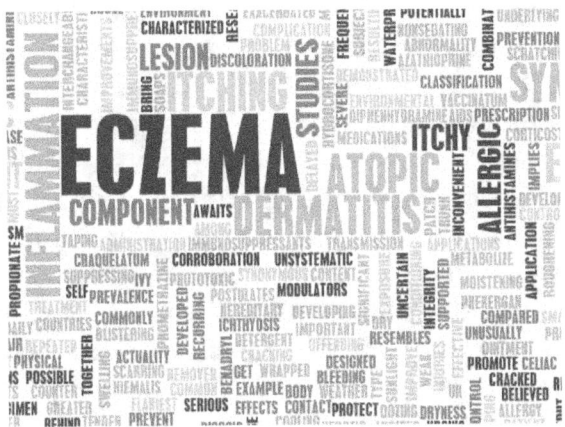

Scientifically speaking, eczema is a general medical term which primarily refers to the inflammation and irritation of the epidermis or the outer layer of the skin. It is initially characterized by the reddening, oozing, weeping, crusting, and drying of the small papules and vesicles of the skin, then later on, you will notice the scaling and pigmentation of the areas.

But basically, in layman's term, it is a medical condition that is commonly displayed as an irritation and inflammation of the skin.

In some conditions, when eczema is still under its development, the affected areas of the skin may look red and elevated with some tiny blisters of the vesicles that contain clear liquid. But when the blisters pop, the fluid will leak out and the area will start to ooze. In chronic or old eczema, however, the affected areas appear to be thickened, elevated, scaly, and very dry. But no matter which part of the skin is affected or how long it has been affected, eczema is almost always itchy and discomfort-causing. Usually rashes on the face, the back portion of the wrists, hands, knees, or feet may appear after the itching starts depending on its type of skin disease condition. However, other areas of the skin may also be affected by this medical condition.

Initially for fair-skinned people, the areas of the skin that is suffering from this condition will appear reddish at first, then it will later on turn brown. For dark-skinned people, the affected areas of the skin will appear darker or lighter, depending on the pigmentation.

But rather than being a specific condition, eczema is actually a group of diseases of the skin that may be related and have similar appearances. There are several types of skin conditions that can initiate the development of eczema.

Here is a list of the various skin diseases that closely resemble each other and are somehow related to eczema:

1. Atopic Dermatitis

Those who have a predisposition to inhalant irritants are most likely to develop atopic dermatitis. This is a condition in which the rashes usually appear on the cheeks, neck, elbows, ankles, and knee creases. It is the most common kind of eczema among many individuals.

2. Stasis Dermatitis

This is a skin condition that is common to those who have poor blood circulation in the veins around the legs. Which is why, characteristically so, the inflammation and irritation often appears on the lower legs.

3. Irritant Dermatitis

When the skin is usually exposed to toxic substances brought about by some cosmetics and other chemicals that are usually directly applied on the skin, rashes may start to appear and irritant dermatitis may likely develop.

4. Seborrheic Eczema

This kind of skin disease is characterized by a rash on the face, scalp, ears, and mid-chest for adults.

Among infants, the rashes may appear weepy and oozy and even exist to be quite more extensive than the other types of skin diseases. There is a high possibility that the rashes would spread all over the infant's body.

5. *Xerotic Eczema*

If you have xerotic eczema, your skin may appear very dry causing it to turn red, crack and eventually ooze. This is also characterized by an overall itch of the body most especially on the shins and arms. Commonly, this is triggered by longer times spent in hot bathes and constant use of harsh soaps most especially during the winter season. Doing so causes the normal water barrier of the skin to be breached.

6. *Pompholyx or Dyshidrotic Eczema*

Pompholyxeczema, which is also known as dyshidrotic eczema, is a common skin disease but this has been poorly understood and seldom given attention. Characteristically, this condition affects the skin around the area of your hands (on the sides of the fingers and palms) and soles of the feet by forming rashes and tiny vesicles with clear fluid inside.

7. *Nummular Eczema*

Nummular eczema is a non-specific term for the scaling, itching, and inflaming of the skin that often looks like coin patches. The affected areas are usually your arms and legs but, at times, the coin-shaped lesions can also spread throughout your torso. This skin disease is usually common among people with very sensitive skin.

Chapter 2 - Bringing About Eczema
Causes And Triggers

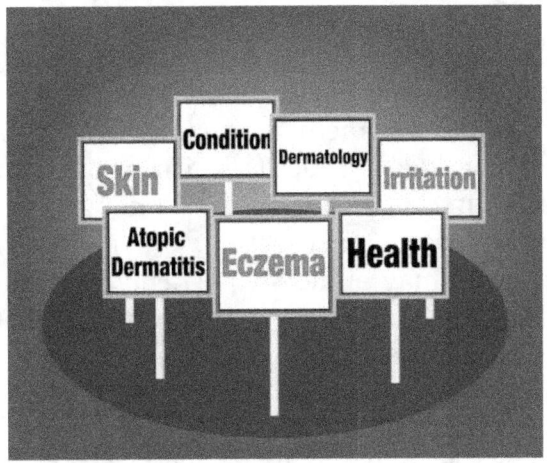

So, you may be asking now:*how does eczema actually develop and cause all the discomfort that are brought about by its manifestations?*

Eczema is basically caused by a similar reaction like that of an allergy and at the same time, it also develops like asthma. Since this disease has many types, the factors that can often cause an allergic reaction on the skin that can in turn lead to this skin disease likewise vary among individuals who have experienced this condition.

To categorize, the causes of this skin disease may either be hereditary or environmental. If eczema or even asthma and hay fever, often runs in your family line, then genetically you are predisposed to its development as well. However, for environmental factors, irritation and inflammation may vary among each individuals' skin reaction. But generally, irritants may either be particulates in the environment. Consider food intake as well as there are a lot of allergens that are contained in foods.

For the particulates, materials, and chemicals being used in the exterior part of the skin, what should be avoided are those that tend to cause irritation and these can include but are not limited to the following:

1. Cosmetics

Aesthetics is very much valued nowadays and with that, the cosmetic industry is also booming and producing more goods to help us look our best.But some perfumes, colognes, make-up, facial creams, lotions and other preserved chemicals that are added to the skin can be irritating and may trigger the appearance of rashes and development of eczema. Pores, especially on the facial area, may easily be breached by chemicals, which is why the application of these products on the skin may cause harmful effects like the development of eczema. So, take extra precaution with what you apply on your skin or better yet, love your own beauty and settle on your natural appearance.

2. Soap and Detergents

When you use too much soap and detergents, they eventually tend to remove the natural oil on your skin and cause it to dry up and become more sensitive to other irritants. Instead of using hard soaps and strong detergents, you can use moisturizers for the body or use hypo allergenic gloves and detergents.Using these willprotect your skin from potential harm, drying up and cracking.

3. Clothing

Of course, you do not have to go naked in order for you to avoid the irritation that some cloth may cause you, but you have to consider the type of cloth you are going to wear for some may trigger the flaring of eczema.

When you go to a thrift store, you perhaps noticed that some clothes are heavily scented and these have been caused by chemicals used by manufacturers especially for heavily printed materials. As much as possible, avoid those. If you are fun of vintage clothes, make sure to examine carefully if those clothes have been cured with chemicals too. You would not want to get yourself harmed in the end, would you?

Cotton and the likes of it that are soft on the skin are safe to use. Fabrics like wool and other rough textured cloths can cause irritation and itchiness on the skin. So to avoid this, better keep cotton and cotton poly fabrics inside your closet.

4. Heat

Excessive exposure to heat can cause your pores to open for sweating. This aggravation may cause drying up and increased sensitivity to other irritants which can later on result to the development of a skin disease that falls under eczema classification. When the sun is at its hottest, be sure to stay indoors.

5. Extreme coldness

While the heat can open your pores, exposing yourself to too much cold can also turn the eczema symptoms on. You have perhaps experienced getting chapped lips. The same thing can happen on your skin when your surrounding gets too cold. Your skin becomes really dry then gets cracked and would begin to itch. During winter season, protective clothing is very important to combat the harsh weather and not only that. You need to moisturize your skin every now and then to keep it from getting dry. The use of natural moisturizers is highly recommended. Always maintain your room's humidity when staying indoors.

6. Hot shower or hot bath

When getting a hot bath may seem relieving, think twice. This can be a trigger too. As the heat can dry your skin up and irritate it. Don't stay too long in the shower. Bath in lukewarm water but do it very quickly.

7. Excessive scrubbing

Scrubbing can cleanse your body as dirt is removed from your skin but using a hard scrub can cause cuts.

8. Air Particulates

Dust, animal dander, pollens, molds, and some other air particulates can also cause the skin to have an allergic reaction and inflammation. This may be hard to avoid because, of course, in order to live we must expose ourselves to air and breathe in oxygen. So the best and most practical way that you can do in order to deal with these irritants is to make sure that you keep your environment clean and well-maintained.

It is important to have plants around in your garden to cleanse the air and absorb dust in the surroundings but make sure you carefully select those plants too so you can avoid those that can potentially cause allergies. Having flowering plants are of course great to add beauty to your surroundings. However, you need to exercise much caution. Inhaling pollens or getting near them can potentially harm your skin.

Exerting effort to beautify your surroundings is never an excuse for you to disregard your health.

9. Food

As also said in the first part of this chapter, foods contain different kinds of allergens and each individual can be allergic with one allergen while others are not. To help you determine which foods you are allergic to, consulting a physician is necessary. See Chapter 5 for an additional discussion about food and what eczema patients should avoid as much as possible.

10. Indoor dusts

Make your home dust-free especially for kids. Rugs and blinds should be cleaned. Bed sheets, pillow cases, and seat covers must be washed well and replaced often, at least once a week as these materials retain much dust that gets into your homes. A general cleaning is proper to keep your family safe at all times. You would not want your kids to suffer later on.

11. Pets

If you have pets at home, carefully observe whether they cause you irritation as well. Especially for those who have access outdoors, your dogs or cats may bring in dust in their fur or pollens as they roam around your garden. If they are excessive shedders, then there is no reason that you would not have cough or asthma attacks especially when their fur would get through your nostrils. Make sure you vacuum carpets and corners of your home well that retain their fur. You may consider leaving your dog with your relatives too or limit their access around the house.

12. Habitual Itch-Scratch Cycle

This is neither a particulate nor a material added on the skin but nevertheless, this potentially causes the worsening of the symptoms of eczema. For when the skin starts to react to irritants, we tend to scratch the itchiness away.

That reaction is pretty normal. The only thing you want is to get rid of the uneasy feeling. However, the itch-scratch cycle can only worsen the condition since it irritates the skin even more and cause it to even develop a wound and bleed furthermore. If this is a habit that you have developed, you may want to try wearing cotton gloves or mittens to avoid wounding and worsening the condition. Instead of scratching, you may also just rub the affected area in order to relieve the itchiness.

13. Stress

Stress may not cause eczema but it can worsen your condition. It is one trigger that has often been disregarded by many. When you get tired and exhausted, your brain gives the signals throughout your body and your skin is not at all exempted from experiencing the same. You will notice your skin losing its moisture and then becoming itchy which will cause you to scratch it. As mentioned earlier, scratching your skin once you get that itchy feeling will make the situation worse as it will cause more soreness and dryness which will in turn make it itchier. Hence the habitual scratching cycle.

There are a lot of ways to improve your overall wellbeing and provide temporarily relief if not totally eliminating stress in your life. Among these are engaging in worthwhile activities that captures your interest, doing meditation and yoga, and a lot more. Take charge of yourself and be in control of your emotions. When life gets too busy and everything seems to take a toll on you, say a little prayer of thanks and think of happy thoughts. Somehow, the thought of something that made you smile would cost you nothing but bring about a great change in your mood and life.

Chapter 3 - Eczema Prevalence Age, Gender, And Race

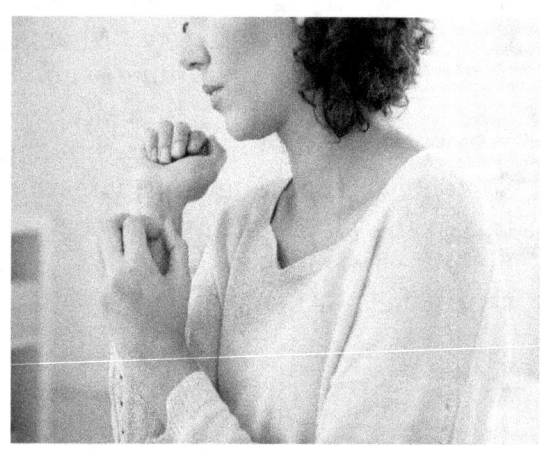

Until now, there are still a substantial number of people with eczema in the United States. This is due to lack of good treatments that could target and eradicate the disease fully. Even in this modern age, there is still too little understanding about the disease itself and the development of effective treatments to fully get rid of the disease is also still ongoing. According to a research conducted by the National Eczema Organization (NEO), there are around

31.6 million who are suffering from eczema in the United States and around 17.8 million of them have moderate to severe cases.

Age

Eczema usually begins in childhood and is carried on by the person up until adulthood. In the survey conducted by the NEO, the prevalence of eczema in children is about 10.7% and 10.2% in adults. It can be drawn from this data that most children still continue to get eczema flare-ups even in their adulthood.

Gender

This medical condition can possibly affect both sexes, but at a peak time in the females' adolescence to adulthood of 15 to 49 years of age, eczema is most likely to appear and attack.

Race

From a survey documented between the years 2000 to 2010, eczema has widely affected many races. The prevalence of the condition among non-Hispanic black children in the United States have increased from 8.6% to 17.1%. For Hispanic children, the prevalence rose from 5% to 9.9%. And from 7.6%, the prevalence among non-Hispanic white children increased to 12.6%.

It can be concluded that eczema actually knows no discrimination, it can affect people of different ages mostly beginning in childhood or infancy stretching up until those children's adult years. It can also affect any gender as well as race— Hispanic or non-Hispanic. Which is why preventive measures should continuously be made and stay applicable to those who are experiencing or have experienced eczema in their early years of life.

Chapter 4 - Natural Home Remedies For Eczema

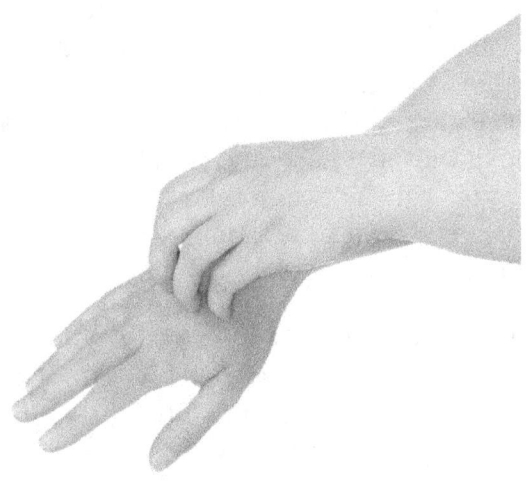

Home is where the healing begins.

If you are among the many individuals across the globe who have been suffering from this condition for your entire life, keep your focus on this chapter as I will be sharing with you some secrets.

Whilethere is no permanent cure for eczema,this condition can however be managed even by simple homemade remedies— you can make use of ingredients within your reach at your pantry or kitchen counters, or even your gardens. The basic thing to do would be to keep your environment clean and remove or replace products that can cause the trigger or exacerbation of the condition. You can avoid using cosmetics especially those that are hard and harsh on the skin or you can also opt for replacements of products, like replacing soaps with moisturizers instead.

Moreover, you do not really have to worry and even look too far for medical products to keep the condition manageable. There is no need to purchase expensive ointments and other products to cure eczema because natural oils, vegetables, and some fruits which you can easily find in your own homes can be used to replace those medicines. This is proof enough that truly your home is where your healing can begin.

Some of these most common home remedies include the following:

1. Milk

You may soak a piece of cotton washcloth in ice-cold milk for around 3 to 5 minutes. Then lay the washcloth on the affected areas on your skin. You can do this for several times during the day as needed. This is to reduce the symptom of itching of the affected areas of the skin.

2. Oatmeal Floats

Excessive use of harsh soaps on your skin can cause it to dry up and become more sensitive to irritants but there can be a more soothing way of bathing. You may have ground oatmeal floats added to your water for bathing. The suspension of the oats on water during your bath can sooth your skin and lessen the itch.

3. Virgin Coconut Oil

You may also apply organic cold-pressed virgin coconut oil to the affected areas of the skin in order to lessen the rash and then on, the itch. You can apply it immediately on skin or by the use of a washcloth soaked in virgin coconut oil. You can choose and do so the process you prefer.

4. Cucumber

You may also cut a whole organic cucumber into thin slices and soak these slices in water for at least two hours. Then, you can filter the water by sifting its large particles from the liquid itself. Soak a piece of washcloth into the filtered liquid and compress the cloth on the affected areas.

5. Chamomile Tea

To eliminate acute symptoms of eczema, you may apply chamomile tea to the affected areas of the skin. But you have to brew it first by steeping the bag for at least 15 minutes in warm water. Then soak a washcloth into the tea and apply to the affected skin areas.

6. Aloe Vera

The aloe vera gel, especially when added with Vitamin E oil, is best for relieving the symptoms of itching and inflaming of eczema. Like applying an ointment, you may simply add and spread the gel on the affected parts of the skin.

7. Carrot Paste

You can make a homemade carrot paste by skinning 3 or 4 medium-sized carrots and boiling them until they are soft enough to mash. Then, mash these carrots until they start to appear like paste. Apply the carrot paste on the affected areas for 15 minutes and rinse the areas with cool water after the application.

8. Tea tree Oil Bath

Mixing a few drops of tea tree oil whenever you take a refreshing bath will help you in dealing with eczema as tea tree oil contains natural antiseptic properties. Incorporating this in your bath will keep your skin from getting infections which will then bring about the triggers.

Chapter 5 - Eat Your Way Out Food Choices For Those With Eczema

Making home remedies for eczema is not the only way to reduce the symptoms that it can bring. Food intake is also a key major factor in managing the skin disease because in some studies, eczema has been found to be a third to two thirds linked with food allergies. Eczema can flare-up from 2 to 24 hours upon the consumption of these foods. Aside from eczema, gastrointestinal discomfort can be experienced as well. But worry no more because by now, you can eat your way out of eczema by knowing which foods to eat and avoid.

What to Avoid

Food can also trigger eczema as some of them can elicit allergic reactions from the body. In order to avoid the flaring of eczema, these foods should also be avoided.

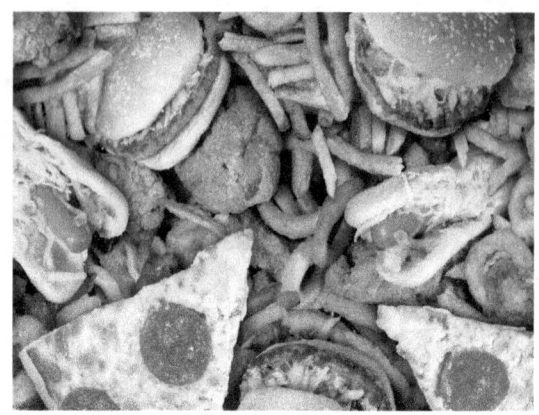

Refined Carbohydrates and Sugar

Consuming food rich in refined carbohydrates and sugar can upset the processing of the essential fatty acids like omega-3. The fighting off of the symptoms of eczema would then be cut off short, thereby prolonging the condition. Foods rich with these substances are: pasta, white rice, cakes, cookies, and lasagna.

Saturated Fats

Food rich in saturated fats can cause the condition to worsen its inflammatory symptom. Packed, processed, and deep-fried foods are very rich in saturated fats and are not good for your health especially when you have eczema. These foods rich in saturated fats are: red meat (pork and beef meat), dairy products like cheese, milk, and butter, junk food, and other deeply fried food.

Protein

Some sources of protein can trigger the flaring up of eczema. Foods like eggs, nuts, seeds, soy products, and chicken are some of the protein-rich triggers.

What to Eat Instead

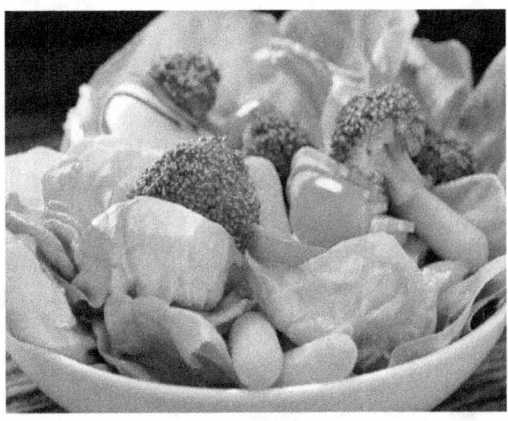

When you have eczema, you will need nutrients that would reduce the inflammation and irritation of the condition. Some of these nutrients are best gained by what you take into your body—that is, food.

Omega-3

Consume foods that are rich in healthy and essential fatty acids like omega 3. Doing so can lessen the allergic reaction brought about by eczema. Omega 3 is rich in amounts in the following foods: walnuts, avocadoes, tuna, mackerel, and salmon among others.

Zinc

This is one of the nutrients that could facilitate the processing of the essential fatty acids and the healing of your skin, diminishing the allergic symptoms of eczema. Taking 30 milligrams of zinc everyday can help you deal with the condition. You can obtain this nutrient from some of these foods: oysters, spinach, and cocoa.

Protein

Lean protein and protein from vegetables are best for the reduction of the symptoms of eczema. Good sources of protein are: potato, broccoli, and corn.

Fiber

Fiber can facilitate the functions of your endocrine system, removing the wastes and toxins from your body and at the same time, cleaning your gut. With its process in the body, it can lessen the chances of food sensitivities. Good sources of fiber are: whole grains, fresh fruits, and most especially, green leafy vegetables.

Water

Like fiber, water can also aid the removal of toxins from the body, reducing the food sensitivities of the body and relieving more work from the kidneys and better fight off with the food allergens.

The key here is to eat a healthy diet and avoid allergy-causing foods since they could trigger or worsen the eczema flare-up. Be a police in what you specifically eat in order for you to keep a distance from eczema.

CONCLUSION

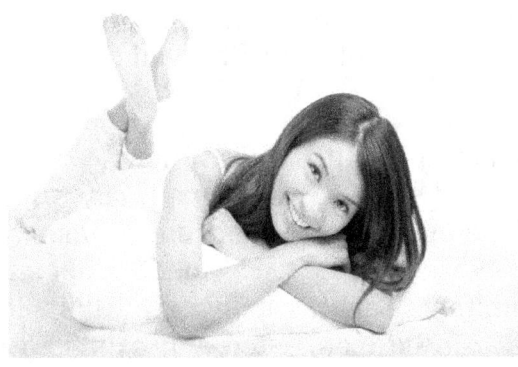

Thank you again for downloading this book!

I hope this book was able to help you to know more about Eczema in order for you to keep it under control through home remedies and natural treatment.

To sum up all the points presented in this book, eczema is a general term for a medical condition of a cluster of skin problems that actually knows no discriminationamong ages, genders, and even races. It is continuously substantially prevalent among the US population due to the lack of information

41

about the condition and knowledge for treatment that could fully eradicate it. Until now, the treatments available for eczema are those that could only eliminate itsattendant symptoms like rashes, reddening, itching, and inflaming.

However, eczema can be very manageable, much like asthma, so there is no need to worry and panic. By simply following the recommended homemade remedies and correct food intake, the symptoms such as itching and inflaming that can be manifested and exhibited by this condition, will surely be reduced.

Some kitchen and home products such as milk, oatmeal, virgin coconut oil, cucumber, chamomile tea, aloe vera, and carrot paste can all be made at home in order to keep the condition under management and reduce the itchiness and inflammation. All these products can be found in common households that most people do not realize they have the treatments right inside their homes and not really in pharmacies.

Correct diet for those with eczema can also help in the avoidance and worsening conditions of the disease. Certain kinds of food are said to cause allergic reactions for some individuals and, thus, later on develop further into a flaring eczema. Knowing exactly what foods to avoid and what to eat instead is very important you are experiencing or when you have experienced eczema for knowing so can help you choose better on what to eat and so you could keep the eczema under control.

Eczema is a common skin disease and it could happen to many people. So, with that, you do not really have to raise your alarms up in wild motions because the treatments are simply right within your reach— at home. Simply by following the instructions correctly as provided in this book, you will be able to make temporary cures for the symptoms of eczema. So, do not worry and start putting eczema under your control.

The next step is to go ahead and make your own treatments for eczema and you will surely worry no more.

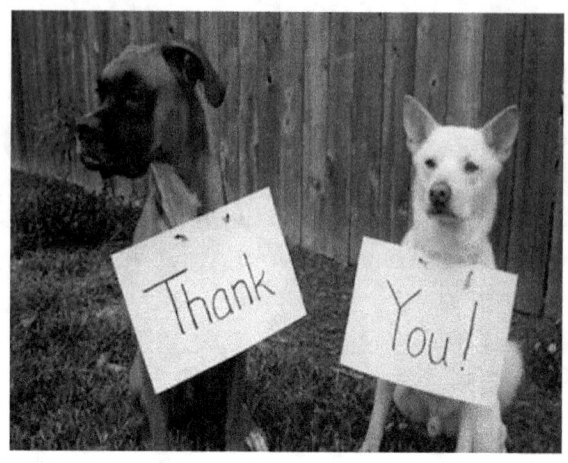

Finally, if you enjoyed this book, then I'd like to ask you for a favor, would you be kind enough to leave a review for this book on Amazon? It'd be greatly appreciated!

Click here to leave a review for this book on Amazon!

Thank you and good luck!

www.ingramcontent.com/pod-product-compliance
Lightning Source LLC
Chambersburg PA
CBHW071143280526
45787CB00003B/1386